ANTI CANDIDA DIET COOKBOOK

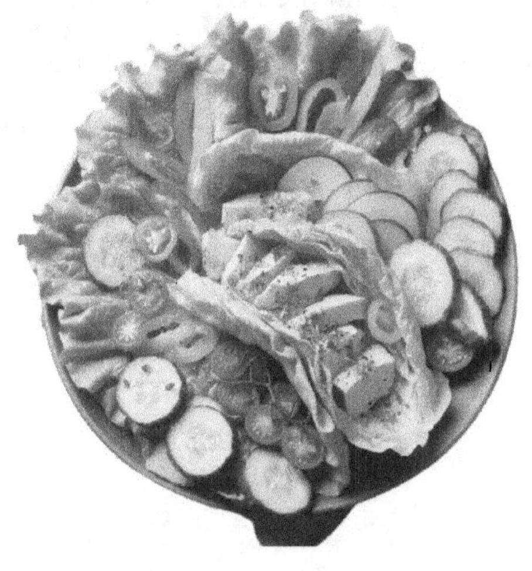

Delicious Anti Candida Recipes for Vibrant Health

LANITA CRUZ

TABLE OF CONTENT

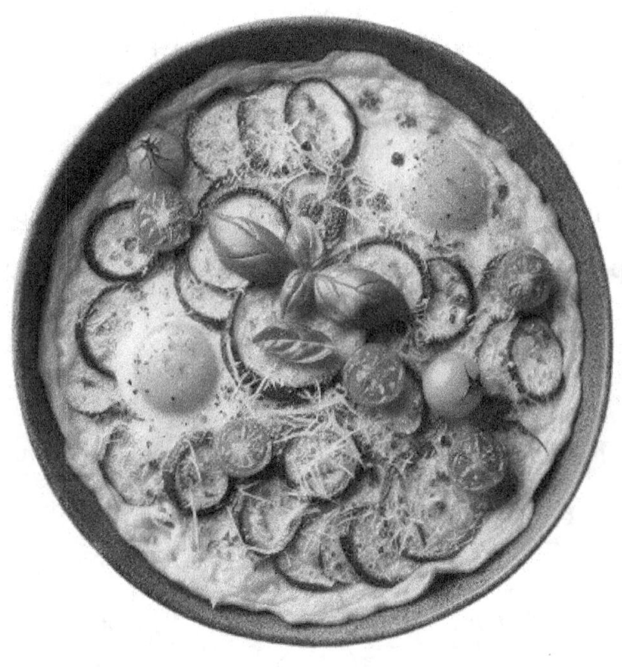

INTRODUCTION

Have you ever experienced unexplained fatigue, digestive woes, brain fog, or stubborn weight gain? If so, you're not alone. Millions of people worldwide struggle with these symptoms, often caused by an overgrowth of a type of yeast called Candida albicans in the gut.

While Candida is naturally present in our digestive system, its overabundance can lead to a condition known as candidiasis, impacting our overall health and well-being.

This book, your essential guide to the Anti-Candida Diet, empowers you to take control of your gut health and reclaim your vibrant life. Forget restrictive fads and confusing information; here, you'll discover a science-backed, practical approach to managing Candida and fostering a thriving gut microbiome.

Through the pages that follow, you'll gain a deep understanding of the Anti-Candida Diet's principles and benefits. We'll explore the foods that nourish your body and starve Candida, equipping you with a comprehensive shopping list and delectable recipes for every meal. From satisfying breakfasts and power-packed lunches to mouthwatering dinners and guilt-free treats, this book provides a culinary adventure that supports your healing journey.

But this is more than just a cookbook; it's a roadmap to lasting gut health. We'll delve into the science behind Candida overgrowth, its impact on your body, and the powerful tools you can wield to achieve balance. You'll also find a 30-day meal plan sample, offering a practical starting point for your Anti-Candida journey.

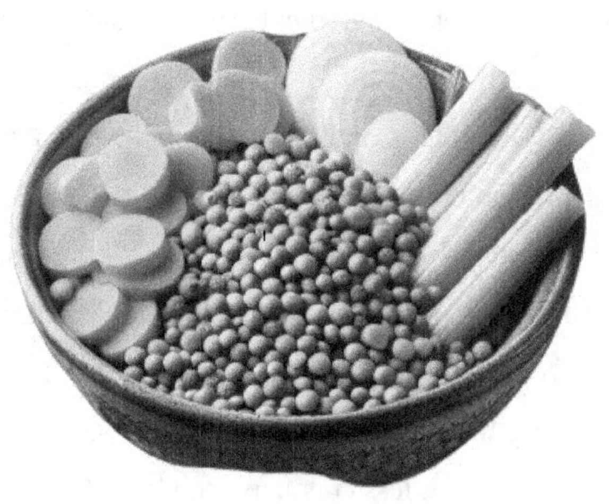

CHAPTER 1

Principles of the Anti-Candida Diet

1. **Elimination of Sugars and Refined Carbohydrates**: The foremost principle involves cutting off the fuel supply for Candida by eliminating sugars and refined carbohydrates. This starves the yeast, hindering its ability to thrive and proliferate in the body.

2. **Incorporation of Antifungal Foods**: Emphasizing the consumption of natural antifungal foods becomes pivotal. Ingredients such as garlic, coconut oil, oregano, and olive oil possess properties that actively combat Candida overgrowth, promoting a balanced internal environment.

3. **Probiotic-rich Foods:** Supporting the body's beneficial bacteria is crucial. Probiotic-rich foods like yogurt, kefir, and fermented vegetables aid in restoring the microbial balance in the gut, creating an environment less conducive to Candida.

4. **Nutrient-Dense, Whole Foods:** A diet centered around nutrient-dense, whole foods ensures that the

body receives essential vitamins and minerals, bolstering the immune system and fostering an environment that discourages Candida growth.

5. **Moderation and Balance:** The principle of moderation extends to all aspects of the diet. Balancing macronutrients, avoiding excessive consumption of certain foods, and maintaining portion control contribute to overall wellness and Candida control.

6. **Hydration:** A well-hydrated body aids in flushing toxins and supporting various physiological functions. Ample water intake is encouraged to promote optimal digestion and discourage Candida proliferation.

7. **Individualized Approach:** Recognizing that you may respond differently to dietary changes, the principles encourage your approach. This involves paying attention to personal reactions to foods and making adjustments based on your needs.

By comprehensively addressing these principles, you can effectively disrupt the Candida cycle, promoting a balanced internal environment conducive to overall health and well-being.

Benefits of the Anti-Candida Diet

1. **Balanced Gut Microbiota:** The Anti-Candida diet fosters a balanced gut microbiota by promoting the growth of beneficial bacteria. This microbial balance is essential for proper digestion, nutrient absorption, and overall immune function.

2. **Increased Energy Levels:** By eliminating sugars and refined carbohydrates that can lead to energy crashes, you often experience more consistent and sustained energy levels throughout the day.

3. **Enhanced Digestive Function:** A diet rich in nutrient-dense, whole foods supports optimal digestive function. This can alleviate symptoms such as bloating, gas, and indigestion often associated with Candida overgrowth.

4. **Improved Mental Clarity:** Reduced consumption of inflammatory foods and the promotion of gut health are linked to improved cognitive function and mental clarity. Many individuals report enhanced focus and reduced brain fog.

5. **Weight Management:** The elimination of processed foods and sugars, coupled with a focus on whole, nutrient-dense foods, supports healthy weight management. This is beneficial not only for physical health but also for reducing stress on the body.

6. **Stronger Immune System**: A well-balanced diet contributes to a stronger immune system. By promoting the growth of beneficial bacteria and reducing the burden of harmful pathogens, the body is better equipped to defend against infections and illnesses.

7. **Alleviation of Candida Symptoms:** Suffering from Candida overgrowth, you often experience symptoms such as recurrent yeast infections, fatigue, and joint pain. The Anti-Candida diet aims to alleviate these symptoms by addressing the root cause of the issue.

8. **Overall Well-being:** Beyond specific health improvements, adhering to the Anti-Candida diet can contribute to a general sense of well-being. You

often report feeling lighter, more energetic, and experiencing a positive impact on their mood.

By highlighting these benefits, the section encourages you to view the Anti-Candida diet not just as a means to address a specific health issue but as a holistic approach to enhancing overall quality of life.

Foods to eat

Non-Starchy Vegetables: Load your plate with a colorful array of non-starchy vegetables such as leafy greens, broccoli, cauliflower, zucchini, and bell peppers. These fiber-rich choices not only provide essential nutrients but also contribute to a balanced gut environment.

Lean Proteins: Prioritize lean protein sources like poultry, fish, eggs, and plant-based proteins such as tofu and legumes. Protein is vital for muscle repair, immune function, and satiety, supporting overall health during the Candida-fighting journey.

Healthy Fats: Incorporate healthy fats like avocados, nuts, seeds, and olive oil into your meals. These fats provide sustained energy, aid in nutrient absorption, and have anti-inflammatory properties, promoting a balanced internal environment.

Herbs and Spices: Enhance the flavors in your recipes by incorporating various herbs and spices. Garlic, oregano, turmeric, and ginger not only add zest but also possess antifungal properties, supporting the body in its battle against Candida overgrowth.

Probiotic-Rich Foods: Include probiotic-rich foods like yogurt, kefir, sauerkraut, and kimchi. These support the growth of beneficial bacteria in the gut, contributing to a healthy microbial balance.

Low-Sugar Fruits: Opt for low-sugar fruits such as berries, green apples, and citrus fruits in moderation. These provide essential vitamins and antioxidants without contributing significantly to sugar levels.

Whole Grains in Moderation: Choose whole grains like quinoa, brown rice, and buckwheat in moderation. While these provide essential nutrients, limiting their intake prevents overconsumption of carbohydrates.

Alternative Sweeteners: Explore alternative sweeteners such as stevia and xylitol sparingly. These can satisfy sweet cravings without promoting Candida growth, as opposed to traditional sugars.

Foods to avoid

Refined Sugars: Steer clear of refined sugars, high-fructose corn syrup, and artificial sweeteners. These provide a fertile ground for Candida overgrowth and contribute to inflammation in the body.

Processed Foods: Eliminate processed foods and snacks that often contain hidden sugars, preservatives, and additives. Opting for whole, unprocessed foods supports the body's natural healing process.

High-Carb Foods: Minimize the consumption of high-carbohydrate foods such as white bread, pasta, and pastries. These rapidly convert to sugar in the body, exacerbating Candida proliferation.

Dairy Products: Temporarily avoid dairy products, as they can be a source of lactose, which may feed Candida. Think about opting for plant-based alternatives, such as almond or coconut milk.

Alcohol: Restrict or eliminate alcohol, as it not only contains sugars but also disrupts the balance of gut flora, promoting conditions favorable for Candida overgrowth.

Fruits High in Sugar: Limit fruits high in natural sugars, such as bananas, grapes, and mangoes. Opt for lower-sugar alternatives to maintain a balanced intake.

Gluten-Containing Grains: Exclude gluten-containing grains like wheat, barley, and rye. Gluten can contribute to inflammation and compromise gut health.

Caffeine: Reduce or eliminate caffeine, as it can overstimulate the nervous system and potentially disrupt the balance of beneficial bacteria in the gut.

Certain Vegetables: Limit the intake of starchy vegetables like potatoes and corn, as they can elevate blood sugar levels.

Mold-Containing Foods: Avoid foods prone to mold, such as aged cheeses, peanuts, and moldy grains. Mold can exacerbate symptoms in individuals with Candida overgrowth.

Comprehensive Shopping List for Anti Candida Diet

Here's a comprehensive shopping list tailored for the Anti-Candida Diet:

Proteins:

- Skinless poultry (chicken, turkey)
- Fish (salmon, trout, mackerel)
- Eggs
- Tofu
- Lentils
- Chickpeas
- Black beans

Non-Starchy Vegetables:

- Leafy greens (spinach, kale, arugula)
- Broccoli
- Cauliflower
- Zucchini
- Bell peppers
- Asparagus
- Cucumber

Healthy Fats:

- Avocados
- Nuts (almonds, walnuts, cashews)
- Seeds (chia seeds, flaxseeds, sunflower seeds)
- Olive oil
- Coconut oil

Herbs and Spices:

- Garlic
- Oregano
- Turmeric
- Ginger
- Cinnamon
- Basil
- Parsley

Probiotic-Rich Foods:

- Greek yogurt (unsweetened)
- Kefir
- Sauerkraut
- Kimchi

Low-Sugar Fruits:

- Berries (strawberries, blueberries, raspberries)
- Green apples
- Citrus fruits (lemons, limes)

Whole Grains (in moderation):

- Quinoa
- Brown rice
- Buckwheat

Alternative Sweeteners (sparingly):

- Stevia
- Xylitol

Beverages:

- Water (plain or infused with lemon)
- Herbal teas (peppermint, chamomile)
- Coconut water

Dairy Alternatives:

- Almond milk
- Coconut milk

Condiments and Flavorings:

- Apple cider vinegar

- Mustard (without added sugars)

- Tamari or coconut aminos, a gluten-free substitute for soy sauce.

Snacks:

- Raw vegetables with guacamole

- Nuts and seeds mix

- Coconut chips (unsweetened)

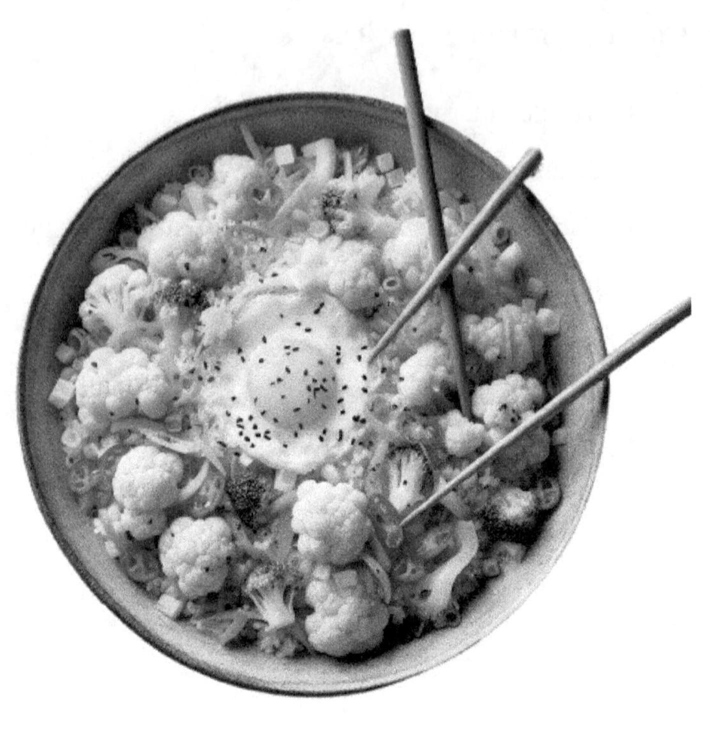

CHAPTER 2

Breakfast Recipes for Anti Candida's Diet

Zucchini Frittata

Preparation Time: 15 minutes

Serves: 4

Ingredients:

- 6 large eggs
- 2 medium zucchinis, grated
- 1/2 cup diced onions
- 1/2 cup cherry tomatoes, halved
- 1/4 cup fresh basil, chopped
- Salt and pepper to taste
- 2 tablespoons olive oil

Nutritional Information: Calories: 180 | Protein: 12g | Carbohydrates: 6g | Fat: 12g

Instructions:

1. Preheat the oven broiler.

2. In a bowl, whisk the eggs and season with salt and pepper.

3. Heat olive oil in an oven-safe skillet over medium heat.

4. Add onions and sauté until translucent, then add grated zucchini and cook until softened.

5. Pour the whisked eggs over the vegetables in the skillet.

6. Sprinkle cherry tomatoes and fresh basil evenly over the eggs.

7. Allow the edges to set for about 3-4 minutes.

8. Transfer the skillet to the preheated broiler and cook for an additional 3-5 minutes until the top is set and slightly golden.

9. Remove from the oven and let it cool for a minute before slicing.

Serving Suggestions:

Serve the Zucchini Frittata slices with a side of fresh salad or avocado for a wholesome and satisfying breakfast.

Sautéed Greens with Poached Eggs

Preparation Time: 10 minutes

Serves: 2

Ingredients:

- 4 large eggs
- 4 cups mixed greens (spinach, kale)
- 1 tablespoon olive oil
- 2 cloves garlic, minced
- Salt and pepper to taste
- Red pepper flakes (optional)

Nutritional Information: Calories: 200 | Protein: 12g | Carbohydrates: 4g | Fat: 16g

Instructions:

1. Heat up olive oil in a large skillet on medium heat.
2. Add minced garlic and sauté until fragrant.
3. Add mixed greens to the skillet and sauté until wilted but still vibrant.
4. Create small wells in the greens and crack eggs into each well.
5. Cover the skillet and poach the eggs for about 3-4 minutes, or until the whites are set but the yolks remain runny.

6. Add salt, pepper, and red pepper flakes as per your preference.

7. Gently transfer the greens and poached eggs to plates.

Serving Suggestions:

Serve the Sautéed Greens with Poached Eggs over a slice of gluten-free toast or alongside sliced avocado for a nutrient-packed breakfast.

Avocado Toast

Preparation Time: 5 minutes

Serves: 2

Ingredients:

- 2 slices gluten-free seed bread
- 1 ripe avocado
- 1 tablespoon lemon juice
- Salt and pepper to taste
- Red pepper flakes (optional)
- Garnish with fresh herbs, such as cilantro or parsley.

Nutritional Information: Calories: 220 | Protein: 5g | Carbohydrates: 20g | Fat: 15g

Instructions:

1. Toast the gluten-free seed bread slices to your liking.
2. While the bread is toasting, mash the ripe avocado in a bowl.
3. Add lemon juice, salt, and pepper to the mashed avocado, mixing well.
4. Once the bread is toasted, spread the mashed avocado evenly over each slice.
5. Sprinkle red pepper flakes if you prefer a hint of heat.
6. Garnish with fresh herbs for added flavor.

Serving Suggestions:

Pair the Avocado Toast with a side of sliced tomatoes or a poached egg for a simple, nutritious, and satisfying breakfast.

Coconut Yogurt Parfait

Preparation Time: 10 minutes

Serves: 2

Ingredients:

- 1 cup unsweetened coconut yogurt
- 1/2 cup mixed berries (strawberries, blueberries, raspberries)
- 2 tablespoons unsweetened shredded coconut
- 1 tablespoon chia seeds
- 1 tablespoon chopped nuts (almonds, walnuts)

Nutritional Information: Calories: 180 | Protein: 5g | Carbohydrates: 15g | Fat: 10g

Instructions:

1. In two serving glasses or bowls, layer half of the coconut yogurt at the bottom.
2. Add a layer of mixed berries on top of the yogurt.
3. Sprinkle a tablespoon of chia seeds evenly over the berries.
4. Add another layer of coconut yogurt.
5. Top with unsweetened shredded coconut and chopped nuts.
6. Repeat the layering process for the second serving.

Serving Suggestions:

Enjoy the Coconut Yogurt Parfait as a refreshing and satisfying breakfast. Customize by adding a drizzle of honey or a sprinkle of cinnamon for extra sweetness and flavor.

Cinnamon Almond Butter Porridge

Preparation Time: 10 minutes

Serves: 2

Ingredients:

- 1 cup almond flour
- 2 cups unsweetened almond milk
- 2 tablespoons almond butter
- 1 teaspoon ground cinnamon
- 1/2 teaspoon vanilla extract
- 1 tablespoon chia seeds (optional)
- Fresh berries for topping

Nutritional Information: Calories: 250 | Protein: 8g | Carbohydrates: 10g | Fat: 20g

Instructions:

1. In a saucepan, combine almond flour, almond milk, almond butter, ground cinnamon, and vanilla extract.
2. Cook over medium heat, stirring constantly until the mixture thickens to a porridge-like consistency.
3. If desired, add chia seeds for additional texture and nutrition.
4. Once the porridge is ready, remove from heat.
5. Divide the porridge into two bowls and top with fresh berries.

Serving Suggestions:

Sprinkle a bit of extra cinnamon on top or add a dollop of coconut yogurt for a delightful twist to your Cinnamon Almond Butter Porridge.

Quinoa Breakfast Bowl

Preparation Time: 15 minutes

Serves: 2

Ingredients:

- 1 cup cooked quinoa
- 1/2 cup unsweetened almond milk
- 1 tablespoon chia seeds
- 1/2 teaspoon vanilla extract
- 1/2 cup mixed berries (strawberries, blueberries)
- 1 tablespoon chopped nuts (e.g., almonds or walnuts)
- 1 tablespoon unsweetened shredded coconut

Nutritional Information: Calories: 220 | Protein: 8g | Carbohydrates: 30g | Fat: 8g

Instructions:

1. In a saucepan, warm the cooked quinoa with almond milk over medium heat.
2. Stir in chia seeds and vanilla extract, allowing the mixture to simmer until it thickens.
3. Once thickened, remove from heat and let it cool slightly.
4. In serving bowls, layer the quinoa mixture with mixed berries.
5. Top with chopped nuts and a sprinkle of unsweetened shredded coconut.

Serving Suggestions:

Drizzle a touch of honey or maple syrup for added sweetness, or add a dollop of Greek yogurt for extra creaminess to your Quinoa Breakfast Bowl.

Gluten-Free Waffles

Preparation Time: 20 minutes

Serves: 4

Ingredients:

- 1 cup gluten-free flour
- 1 teaspoon baking powder
- 1/2 teaspoon baking soda
- 1/4 teaspoon salt
- 2 large eggs
- 1 cup unsweetened almond milk
- 2 tablespoons coconut oil, melted
- 1 tablespoon maple syrup (optional)
- Fresh berries for topping

Nutritional Information: Calories: 180 | Protein: 4g | Carbohydrates: 25g | Fat: 8g

Instructions:

1. Begin by preheating your waffle iron following the guidance provided by the manufacturer.
2. In a large mixing bowl, whisk together gluten-free flour, baking powder, baking soda, and salt.
3. In a separate bowl, beat the eggs and then add almond milk, melted coconut oil, and maple syrup (if using).
4. Combine the wet ingredients with the dry ingredients and stir until thoroughly mixed.
5. Grease the waffle iron with a small amount of coconut oil.
6. Pour the batter onto the preheated waffle iron and cook according to the appliance instructions.
7. Once cooked, remove the waffles and top with fresh berries.

Serving Suggestions:

Serve the Gluten-Free Waffles with a dollop of coconut yogurt or a drizzle of almond butter for a delightful and wholesome breakfast.

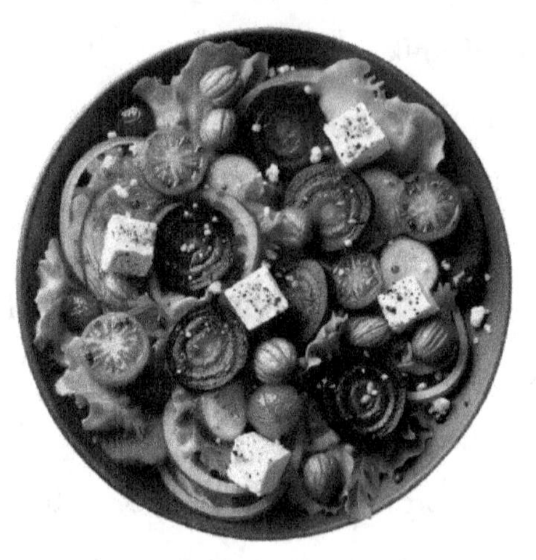

CHAPTER 3

Lunch Recipes for Anti Candida's Diet

Cauliflower Fried Rice

Preparation Time: 20 minutes

Serves: 4

Ingredients:

- 1 medium-sized cauliflower, grated
- 2 cups of assorted vegetables, including carrots, peas, and corn
- 1 cup diced tofu or cooked chicken (optional)
- 3 eggs, beaten
- 3 tablespoons coconut oil
- 2 tablespoons tamari (gluten-free soy sauce)
- 1 teaspoon sesame oil
- 1 teaspoon grated ginger
- 2 cloves garlic, minced
- Salt and pepper to taste
- Garnish with green onions and sesame seeds for added visual appeal.

Nutritional Information: Calories: 180 | Protein: 10g | Carbohydrates: 10g | Fat: 12g

Instructions:

1. In a large skillet, heat coconut oil over medium heat.
2. Add grated cauliflower and sauté until it starts to turn golden brown.
3. Push cauliflower to the side and add a bit more oil. Transfer the beaten eggs into the pan and scramble until they are fully cooked.
4. Add diced tofu or cooked chicken (if using) and mixed vegetables to the skillet. Cook until vegetables are tender.
5. Mix in tamari, sesame oil, grated ginger, and minced garlic. Stir well to combine.
6. Add salt and pepper to taste, seasoning the dish to your liking.
7. Garnish with chopped green onions and sesame seeds before serving.

Serving Suggestions:

Serve Cauliflower Fried Rice as a standalone dish or as a side to grilled chicken or shrimp for a complete and satisfying meal.

Turkey Lettuce Wraps

Preparation Time: 15 minutes

Serves: 4

Ingredients:

- 1 lb ground turkey
- 1 tablespoon coconut oil
- Diced bell peppers, a total of one cup, with a blend of colors.
- 1 cup shredded carrots
- 1/2 cup chopped water chestnuts
- 3 tablespoons tamari (gluten-free soy sauce)
- 1 tablespoon rice vinegar
- 1 teaspoon sesame oil
- 1 teaspoon grated ginger

- 2 cloves garlic, minced
- Iceberg or butter lettuce leaves for wrapping
- Sesame seeds for garnish

Nutritional Information: Calories: 220 | Protein: 18g | Carbohydrates: 8g | Fat: 12g

Instructions:

1. In a large skillet, heat coconut oil over medium heat.
2. Add ground turkey and cook until browned, breaking it apart with a spatula.
3. Add diced bell peppers, shredded carrots, and water chestnuts to the skillet. Sauté until vegetables are tender.
4. In a small bowl, mix tamari, rice vinegar, sesame oil, grated ginger, and minced garlic.
5. Pour the sauce over the turkey and vegetable mixture. Stir well to combine.
6. Simmer for a few minutes until the flavors meld together.
7. Spoon the turkey mixture onto individual lettuce leaves.

8. Garnish with sesame seeds before serving.

Serving Suggestions:

Serve Turkey Lettuce Wraps with a side of cauliflower rice or enjoy them on their own for a light and flavorful lunch.

Greek Salad with Grilled Chicken

Preparation Time: 25 minutes

Serves: 2

Ingredients:

- 2 boneless, skinless chicken breasts
- 1 tablespoon olive oil
- 1 teaspoon dried oregano
- Salt and pepper to taste
- 4 cups mixed greens (lettuce, spinach)
- 1 cup cherry tomatoes, halved
- 1 cucumber, sliced
- 1/2 red onion, thinly sliced
- 1/2 cup Kalamata olives, pitted
- 1/2 cup crumbled feta cheese

- Greek dressing (olive oil, red wine vinegar, dried oregano)

Nutritional Information: Calories: 380 | Protein: 30g | Carbohydrates: 15g | Fat: 22g

Instructions:

1. Get the grill or grill pan ready by preheating it to medium-high heat.
2. Rub chicken breasts with olive oil, dried oregano, salt, and pepper.
3. Grill chicken for about 6-7 minutes per side or until fully cooked.
4. In a large bowl, combine mixed greens, cherry tomatoes, cucumber, red onion, Kalamata olives, and feta cheese.
5. Slice grilled chicken and place on top of the salad.
6. In a small bowl, whisk together olive oil, red wine vinegar, and dried oregano to make the Greek dressing.
7. Drizzle the dressing over the salad and toss gently to combine.

Serving Suggestions:

Enjoy Greek Salad with Grilled Chicken as a satisfying and protein-packed lunch. Serve with a side of tzatziki sauce and a slice of gluten-free bread if desired.

Zucchini Noodles with Pesto

Preparation Time: 15 minutes

Serves: 2

Ingredients:

- 4 medium-sized zucchini, spiralized into noodles
- 1 cup cherry tomatoes, halved
- 1/2 cup pine nuts
- 2 cups fresh basil leaves
- 2 cloves garlic
- 1/2 cup nutritional yeast
- 1/2 cup extra-virgin olive oil
- Salt and pepper to taste
- Lemon zest for garnish

Nutritional Information: Calories: 280 | Protein: 10g | Carbohydrates: 14g | Fat: 22g

Instructions:

1. Spiralize zucchini into noodles using a spiralizer or julienne peeler.

2. In a food processor, combine pine nuts, basil, garlic, and nutritional yeast. Pulse until finely chopped.

3. With the food processor running, slowly drizzle in the olive oil until the pesto reaches a smooth consistency.

4. Season the pesto with salt and pepper to taste.

5. In a large skillet, lightly sauté zucchini noodles until just tender, about 2-3 minutes.

6. Toss zucchini noodles with cherry tomatoes and the prepared pesto until well coated.

7. Serve immediately, garnished with lemon zest.

Serving Suggestions:

Zucchini Noodles with Pesto can be enjoyed on its own or paired with grilled chicken or shrimp for added protein. Sprinkle extra nutritional yeast for a cheesy flavor if desired.

Millet & Grilled Vegetable Salad

Preparation Time: 30 minutes

Serves: 4

Ingredients:

- 1 cup millet, cooked and cooled
- 2 zucchinis, sliced lengthwise
- 1 eggplant, sliced
- 1 red bell pepper, sliced
- 1 yellow bell pepper, sliced
- 1 cup cherry tomatoes, halved
- 1/2 cup crumbled goat cheese (optional)
- 1/4 cup fresh basil, chopped
- 3 tablespoons balsamic vinegar
- 2 tablespoons extra-virgin olive oil
- Salt and pepper to taste

Nutritional Information: Calories: 280 | Protein: 8g | Carbohydrates: 40g | Fat: 10g

Instructions:

1. Cook millet according to package instructions and let it cool to room temperature.
2. Preheat your grill or grill pan, ensuring it reaches medium-high heat.

3. Grill zucchini, eggplant, and bell peppers until tender and slightly charred.

4. In a large bowl, combine cooked millet, grilled vegetables, cherry tomatoes, and crumbled goat cheese (if using).

5. In a small bowl, whisk together balsamic vinegar, olive oil, salt, and pepper.

6. Drizzle the dressing over the salad and toss gently to combine.

7. Garnish with fresh basil before serving.

Serving Suggestions:

Millet & Grilled Vegetable Salad can be served warm or chilled. Enjoy it as a standalone dish or alongside grilled chicken or fish for a wholesome lunch.

Salmon and Avocado Lettuce Wraps

Preparation Time: 20 minutes

Serves: 2

Ingredients:

- 2 salmon fillets
- 1 tablespoon olive oil

- 1 teaspoon lemon zest
- Salt and pepper to taste
- 4 large lettuce leaves (butter or iceberg)
- 1 avocado, sliced
- 1/2 cucumber, thinly sliced
- 1/4 cup red onion, finely sliced
- Fresh dill for garnish

Nutritional Information: Calories: 300 | Protein: 20g | Carbohydrates: 10g | Fat: 20g

Instructions:

1. Preheat the oven to 400°F (200°C).
2. Place salmon fillets on a baking sheet, drizzle with olive oil, sprinkle with lemon zest, salt, and pepper.
3. Bake for 12-15 minutes or until salmon is cooked through and flakes easily.
4. While the salmon is baking, prepare the lettuce wraps by laying out the lettuce leaves.
5. Once the salmon is cooked, flake it with a fork.
6. Assemble the wraps by placing salmon, sliced avocado, cucumber, and red onion on each lettuce leaf.

7. Garnish with fresh dill.

Serving Suggestions:

Serve Salmon and Avocado Lettuce Wraps with a side of lemon wedges and a light vinaigrette dressing for a refreshing and protein-packed lunch.

Stuffed Bell Peppers

Preparation Time: 40 minutes

Serves: 4

Ingredients:

- 4 large bell peppers, each halved and seeds extracted.
- 1 lb ground turkey or chicken
- 1 cup cauliflower rice
- 1 cup diced tomatoes
- 1/2 cup diced onions
- 2 cloves garlic, minced
- 1 teaspoon dried oregano
- 1 teaspoon ground cumin
- Salt and pepper to taste
- 1 cup tomato sauce
- 1/2 cup shredded dairy-free cheese (optional)

- Fresh parsley for garnish

Nutritional Information: Calories: 320 | Protein: 25g | Carbohydrates: 20g | Fat: 15g

Instructions:

1. Preheat the oven to 375°F (190°C).
2. In a skillet, cook ground turkey or chicken until browned. Drain excess fat.
3. Add diced onions and garlic to the skillet. Sauté until onions are translucent.
4. Stir in cauliflower rice, diced tomatoes, dried oregano, ground cumin, salt, and pepper. Cook for an additional 5 minutes.
5. Place bell pepper halves in a baking dish.
6. Stuff each pepper half with the turkey or chicken mixture.
7. Pour tomato sauce over the stuffed peppers.
8. Optionally, sprinkle dairy-free cheese on top.
9. Cover with foil and bake for 25-30 minutes.
10. Garnish with fresh parsley before serving.

Serving Suggestions:

Serve Stuffed Bell Peppers with a side of green salad or steamed vegetables for a wholesome and satisfying lunch.

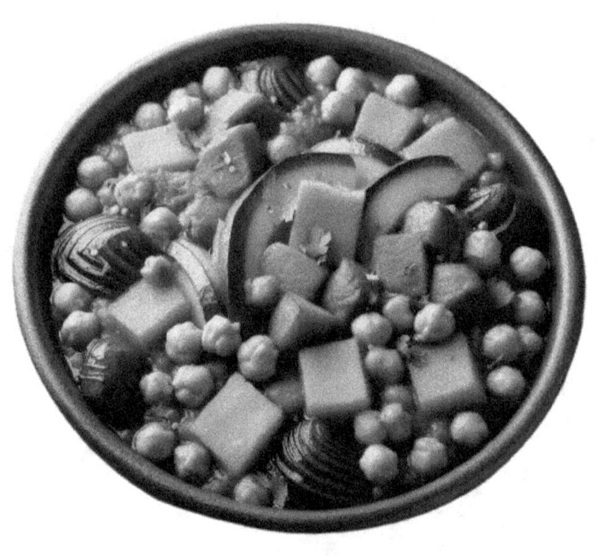

CHAPTER 4

Dinner Recipes for Anti Candida's Diet

Baked Cod with Lemon and Herbs

Preparation Time: 20 minutes

Serves: 4

Ingredients:

- 4 cod fillets
- 2 tablespoons olive oil
- 2 tablespoons fresh lemon juice
- 1 teaspoon lemon zest
- 2 cloves garlic, minced
- 1 teaspoon dried oregano
- 1 teaspoon dried thyme
- Salt and pepper to taste
- Fresh parsley for garnish

Nutritional Information: Calories: 180 | Protein: 25g | Carbohydrates: 1g | Fat: 9g

Instructions:

1. Preheat the oven to 400°F (200°C).
2. Pat the cod fillets dry with a paper towel and place them in a baking dish.
3. In a small bowl, whisk together olive oil, lemon juice, lemon zest, minced garlic, dried oregano, dried thyme, salt, and pepper.
4. Pour the lemon and herb mixture over the cod fillets, ensuring they are well-coated.
5. Bake in the preheated oven for 15-18 minutes or until the cod flakes easily with a fork.
6. Garnish with fresh parsley before serving.

Serving Suggestions:

Serve Baked Cod with Lemon and Herbs with a side of steamed vegetables or a light salad for a wholesome and flavorful dinner. Pair it with quinoa or cauliflower rice for a complete meal.

Chicken Soup

Preparation Time: 30 minutes

Serves: 6

Ingredients:

- One pound of boneless, skinless chicken breasts, cubed.
- 1 tablespoon olive oil
- 1 onion, diced
- 2 carrots, sliced
- 2 celery stalks, chopped
- 3 cloves garlic, minced
- 8 cups chicken broth (low-sodium)
- 1 teaspoon dried thyme
- 1 teaspoon dried rosemary
- 1 bay leaf
- Salt and pepper to taste
- Fresh parsley for garnish

Nutritional Information: Calories: 180 | Protein: 20g | Carbohydrates: 10g | Fat: 7g

Instructions:

1. Start by heating olive oil in a large pot over medium heat; proceed to cook cubed chicken until it turns brown.

2. Add diced onion, sliced carrots, chopped celery, and minced garlic. Sauté until vegetables are tender.

3. Pour in chicken broth and add dried thyme, dried rosemary, bay leaf, salt, and pepper.

4. Bring the soup to a boil, then reduce heat and let it simmer for 20-25 minutes.

5. Remove the bay leaf and discard.

6. Garnish with fresh parsley before serving.

Serving Suggestions:

Enjoy Chicken Soup as a comforting dinner. Serve with a side of gluten-free crackers or a slice of almond flour bread for a satisfying meal.

Cauliflower Hummus

Preparation Time: 15 minutes

Serves: 8

Ingredients:

- 1 medium-sized cauliflower, florets only
- 3 tablespoons tahini
- 2 cloves garlic, minced
- 1/4 cup olive oil

- 2 tablespoons lemon juice

- 1 teaspoon ground cumin

- Salt and pepper to taste

- Paprika for garnish

- Fresh parsley for garnish

Nutritional Information: Calories: 70 | Protein: 2g | Carbohydrates: 4g | Fat: 6g

Instructions:

1. Steam or boil cauliflower florets until very tender.

2. In a food processor, combine steamed cauliflower, tahini, minced garlic, olive oil, lemon juice, ground cumin, salt, and pepper.

3. Blend until smooth and creamy.

4. Taste and adjust seasonings as needed.

5. Transfer the cauliflower hummus to a serving bowl.

6. Drizzle with additional olive oil, sprinkle paprika, and garnish with fresh parsley.

Serving Suggestions:

Serve Cauliflower Hummus with vegetable sticks, gluten-free crackers, or as a side to grilled chicken or fish for a low-carb and nutritious dinner option.

Taco Salad

Preparation Time: 20 minutes

Serves: 4

Ingredients:

- 1 lb ground turkey
- 1 tablespoon olive oil
- 1 onion, diced
- 1 bell pepper, diced
- 1 teaspoon ground cumin
- 1 teaspoon chili powder
- 1/2 teaspoon paprika
- 1/2 teaspoon garlic powder
- Salt and pepper to taste
- 4 cups mixed salad greens
- 1 cup cherry tomatoes, halved
- 1 avocado, sliced
- 1/2 cup dairy-free cheese, shredded

- 1/4 cup fresh cilantro, chopped

- Lime wedges for serving

Nutritional Information: Calories: 320 | Protein: 20g | Carbohydrates: 15g | Fat: 20g

Instructions:

1. Heat olive oil in a skillet over medium heat, then sauté diced onion and bell pepper until they become tender.

2. Add ground turkey, ground cumin, chili powder, paprika, garlic powder, salt, and pepper. Cook until turkey is browned.

3. In a large bowl, assemble the salad by layering mixed greens, cherry tomatoes, sliced avocado, and the cooked turkey mixture.

4. Top with dairy-free cheese and chopped cilantro.

5. Present with lime wedges alongside for added zest..

Serving Suggestions:

Taco Salad is delicious on its own, or you can enjoy it with a dollop of dairy-free sour cream or a scoop of cauliflower rice for a complete meal.

Paprika roasted cabbage wedges

Preparation Time: 25 minutes

Serves: 4

Ingredients:

- A large green cabbage, segmented into wedges
- 3 tablespoons olive oil
- 2 teaspoons smoked paprika
- 1 teaspoon garlic powder
- 1 teaspoon onion powder
- 1/2 teaspoon dried thyme
- Salt and pepper to taste
- Fresh parsley for garnish

Nutritional Information: Calories: 90 | Protein: 2g | Carbohydrates: 10g | Fat: 6g

Instructions:

1. Preheat the oven to 400°F (200°C).
2. Place cabbage wedges on a baking sheet.

3. In a small bowl, whisk together olive oil, smoked paprika, garlic powder, onion powder, dried thyme, salt, and pepper.

4. Brush the paprika mixture over each cabbage wedge, ensuring they are well-coated.

5. Roast in the preheated oven for 20-25 minutes or until the edges are crispy and golden.

6. Garnish with fresh parsley before serving.

Serving Suggestions:

Paprika Roasted Cabbage Wedges can be served as a flavorful side dish alongside grilled chicken or fish. Pair it with a dollop of dairy-free yogurt or a squeeze of lemon for added zest.

Lamb and Buckwheat Meatballs

Preparation Time: 30 minutes

Serves: 6

Ingredients:

- 1 lb ground lamb
- 1 cup cooked buckwheat
- 1 onion, finely chopped

- 2 cloves garlic, minced

- 1 teaspoon dried oregano

- 1 teaspoon ground cumin

- Salt and pepper to taste

- 1/4 cup fresh mint, chopped

- 1/4 cup fresh parsley, chopped

- 1 egg, beaten

- Olive oil for cooking

Nutritional Information: Calories: 280 | Protein: 15g | Carbohydrates: 15g | Fat: 18g

Instructions:

1. In a large bowl, combine ground lamb, cooked buckwheat, chopped onion, minced garlic, dried oregano, ground cumin, salt, and pepper.

2. Add fresh mint, fresh parsley, and beaten egg to the mixture. Mix until well combined.

3. Mold the mixture into meatballs, each measuring approximately 1 inch in diameter.

4. Heat up olive oil in a skillet over medium heat.

5. Cook the meatballs in batches until browned on all sides and cooked through, about 8-10 minutes.

6. Place cooked meatballs on a plate lined with paper towels to absorb excess oil.

Serving Suggestions:

Serve Lamb and Buckwheat Meatballs over a bed of cauliflower rice or alongside a fresh green salad for a hearty and satisfying dinner.

Cabbage Rolls with Turkey and Cauliflower Rice

Preparation Time: 40 minutes

Serves: 4

Ingredients:

- 8 large cabbage leaves
- 1 lb ground turkey
- 1 cup cauliflower rice
- 1 onion, diced
- 2 cloves garlic, minced
- 1 teaspoon dried thyme
- 1 teaspoon paprika
- Salt and pepper to taste

- 1 cup sugar-free tomato sauce

- Fresh parsley for garnish

Nutritional Information: Calories: 280 | Protein: 20g | Carbohydrates: 15g | Fat: 14g

Instructions:

1. Preheat the oven to 375°F (190°C).

2. Heat a substantial pot of water until it reaches a boiling point. Add cabbage leaves and cook for 2-3 minutes or until softened. Drain and set aside.

3. In a skillet, cook ground turkey until browned. Drain excess fat.

4. Add diced onion, minced garlic, dried thyme, paprika, salt, and pepper to the skillet. Sauté until onions are translucent.

5. Stir in cauliflower rice and cook for an additional 5 minutes.

6. Place a spoonful of the turkey mixture onto each cabbage leaf. Roll the leaves and place them seam side down in a baking dish.

7. Pour sugar-free tomato sauce over the cabbage rolls.

8. Bake in the preheated oven for 25-30 minutes or until the rolls are heated through.

9. Garnish with fresh parsley before serving.

Serving Suggestions:

Serve Cabbage Rolls with Turkey and Cauliflower Rice with a side of steamed vegetables or a light salad for a delicious and satisfying dinner.

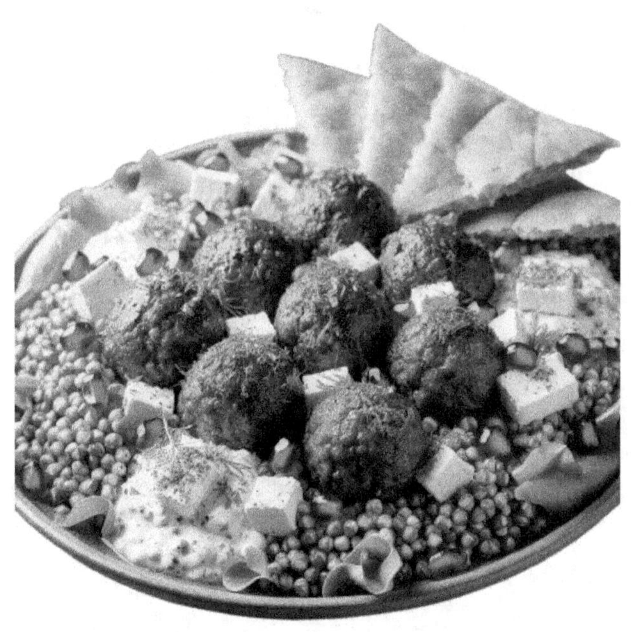

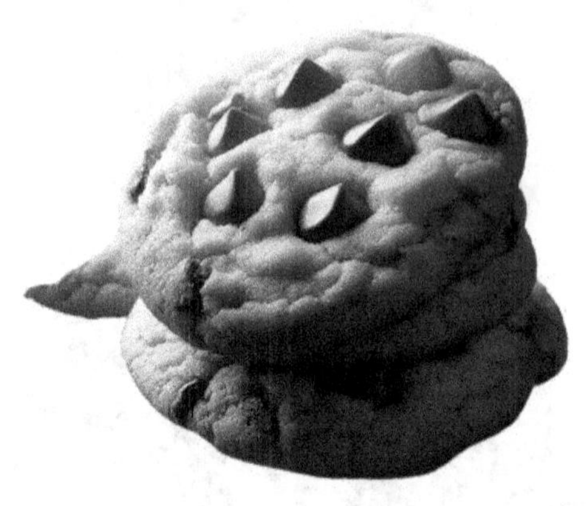

CHAPTER 5

Desserts and Snacks Recipes for Anti Candida's Diet

Coconut Flour Chocolate Chip Cookies

Preparation Time: 25 minutes

Makes: 12 cookies

Ingredients:

- 1/2 cup coconut flour
- 1/4 cup coconut oil, melted
- 1/4 cup sugar-free sweetener (like erythritol)
- 2 eggs
- 1 teaspoon vanilla extract
- 1/4 teaspoon baking soda
- Pinch of salt
- 1/3 cup sugar-free chocolate chips

Nutritional Information: Calories: 90 | Protein: 2g | Carbohydrates: 6g | Fat: 7g

Instructions:

1. Preheat the oven to 350°F (175°C) and cover a baking sheet with parchment paper.

2. In a bowl, whisk together coconut flour, melted coconut oil, sugar-free sweetener, eggs, vanilla extract, baking soda, and a pinch of salt until well combined.

3. Fold in sugar-free chocolate chips.

4. Scoop tablespoon-sized portions of the dough and roll into balls. Place them on the prepared baking sheet, pressing each cookie down slightly.

5. Bake in the preheated oven for 12-15 minutes or until the edges are golden brown.

6. Allow the cookies to cool on the baking sheet for 5 minutes before transferring them to a wire rack to cool completely.

Serving Suggestions:

Enjoy Coconut Flour Chocolate Chip Cookies with a cup of herbal tea or unsweetened almond milk for a delightful and guilt-free snack.

Cinnamon Almond Butter Porridge

Preparation Time: 10 minutes

Serves: 2

Ingredients:

- 1 cup almond flour
- 2 cups unsweetened almond milk
- 2 tablespoons almond butter
- 1 teaspoon ground cinnamon
- 1/2 teaspoon vanilla extract
- Sugar-free sweetener to taste (optional)
- Sliced almonds for garnish (optional)

Nutritional Information: Calories: 300 | Protein: 10g | Carbohydrates: 8g | Fat: 25g

Instructions:

1. In a saucepan, whisk together almond flour and almond milk over medium heat until well combined.
2. Stir in almond butter, ground cinnamon, and vanilla extract.
3. Continue to cook, stirring frequently, until the porridge thickens to your desired consistency.
4. If desired, add sugar-free sweetener to taste.

5. Once the porridge is ready, remove from heat and let it sit for a minute to thicken further.

6. Serve the porridge in bowls, garnished with sliced almonds if desired.

Serving Suggestions:

Cinnamon Almond Butter Porridge can be enjoyed as a warm and comforting breakfast or a satisfying dessert alternative. Pair it with fresh berries for added sweetness and a burst of color.

Turmeric Golden Milk Smoothie

Preparation Time: 5 minutes

Serves: 2

Ingredients:

- 1 cup unsweetened almond milk
- 1 frozen banana
- 1/2 teaspoon ground turmeric
- 1/4 teaspoon ground ginger
- 1/4 teaspoon ground cinnamon
- 1 tablespoon chia seeds
- 1 teaspoon coconut oil

- Sugar-free sweetener to taste (optional)
- Ice cubes (optional)

Nutritional Information: Calories: 150 | Protein: 3g | Carbohydrates: 20g | Fat: 7g

Instructions:

1. In a blender, combine almond milk, frozen banana, ground turmeric, ground ginger, ground cinnamon, chia seeds, and coconut oil.
2. Blend until smooth and creamy.
3. Taste the smoothie and add sugar-free sweetener if desired.
4. If a colder consistency is preferred, add ice cubes and blend again until well combined.
5. Pour the smoothie into glasses and serve right away.

Serving Suggestions:

Enjoy the Turmeric Golden Milk Smoothie as a nutritious and anti-inflammatory snack or breakfast. It's a refreshing option to incorporate the benefits of turmeric into your diet.

Vanilla Coconut Macaroons

Preparation Time: 20 minutes

Makes: 12 macaroons

Ingredients:

- 2 cups shredded unsweetened coconut
- 1/2 cup coconut flour
- 1/4 cup coconut oil, melted
- 1/4 cup sugar-free sweetener (like erythritol)
- 2 large eggs
- 1 teaspoon vanilla extract
- Pinch of salt

Nutritional Information: Calories: 90 | Protein: 2g | Carbohydrates: 5g | Fat: 7g

Instructions:

1. Begin by heating the oven to 350°F (175°C) and covering a baking sheet with parchment paper.
2. In a large bowl, combine shredded coconut, coconut flour, melted coconut oil, sugar-free sweetener, eggs, vanilla extract, and a pinch of salt. Mix until well combined.

3. Using a cookie scoop or your hands, form the mixture into 12 evenly sized macaroons and place them on the prepared baking sheet.

4. Bake in the preheated oven for 12-15 minutes or until the edges are golden brown.

5. Allow the macaroons to cool on the baking sheet for 5 minutes before transferring them to a wire rack to cool completely.

Serving Suggestions:

Vanilla Coconut Macaroons make for a delightful dessert or snack. Pair them with a cup of herbal tea or enjoy them on their own for a sweet and satisfying treat.

Strawberry Smoothie Jell-O

Preparation Time: 15 minutes (plus chilling time)

Serves: 4

Ingredients:

- 2 cups fresh strawberries, hulled and halved
- 1 cup unsweetened almond milk
- 1 tablespoon chia seeds
- 1 teaspoon vanilla extract

- Sugar-free sweetener to taste (optional)
- 2 envelopes unflavored gelatin
- 1/4 cup cold water
- 1/2 cup boiling water

Nutritional Information: Calories: 40 | Protein: 1g | Carbohydrates: 7g | Fat: 1g

Instructions:

1. In a blender, combine fresh strawberries, almond milk, chia seeds, vanilla extract, and sugar-free sweetener if desired. Blend until smooth.
2. In a small bowl, sprinkle gelatin over cold water and let it sit for a minute.
3. Add boiling water to the gelatin mixture and stir until completely dissolved.
4. Pour the gelatin mixture into the blender with the strawberry mixture and blend again until well combined.
5. Pour the mixture into individual serving glasses or molds.
6. Refrigerate for at least 4 hours or until the Jell-O is set.

Serving Suggestions:

Serve Strawberry Smoothie Jell-O chilled as a refreshing and guilt-free dessert or snack. Top with a few sliced strawberries or a dollop of coconut cream for added indulgence.

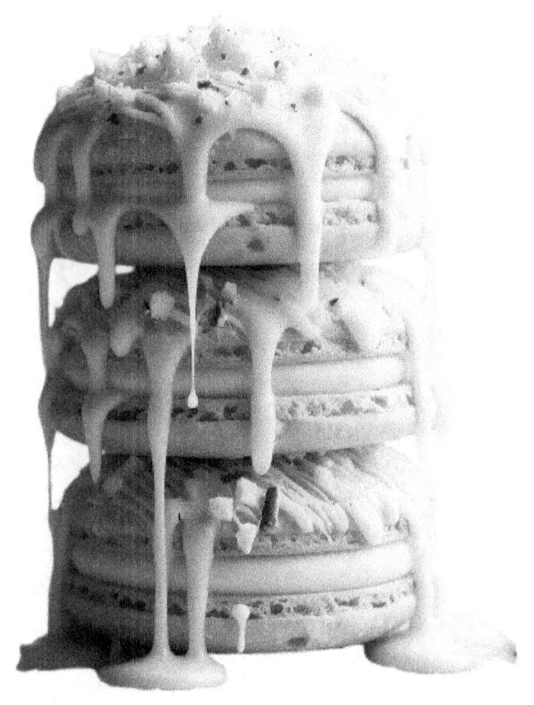

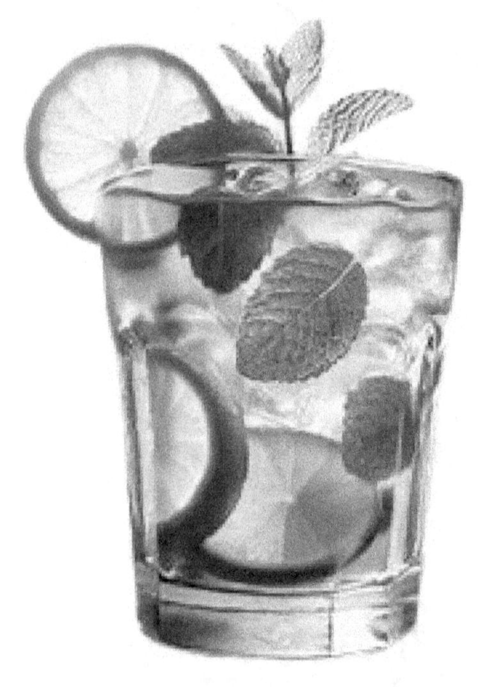

CHAPTER 6

Beverages/Drinks Recipes for Anti-Candida Diet

Moringa Tea

Preparation Time: 10 minutes

Serves: 2

Ingredients:

- 2 teaspoons moringa powder
- 2 cups hot water
- 1 tablespoon lemon juice
- Stevia or another sugar-free sweetener to taste (optional)

Nutritional Information: Calories: 5 | Protein: 1g | Carbohydrates: 1g | Fat: 0g

Instructions:

1. In a teapot, combine moringa powder and hot water. Allow it to steep for 5 minutes.

2. Strain the moringa tea into cups, discarding any residue.

3. Add lemon juice and sweeten with stevia if desired.

4. Stir well and serve hot.

Serving Suggestions:

Enjoy Moringa Tea as a refreshing and nutrient-packed beverage. Pair it with a slice of lemon or a handful of nuts for a light and wholesome snack.

Kombucha

Preparation Time: 7-14 days (fermentation time)

Serves: Varies

Ingredients:

- 1 SCOBY (Symbiotic Culture Of Bacteria and Yeast)
- 4 black or green tea bags
- 1 cup sugar (for feeding the SCOBY)
- Filtered water
- Flavoring options: ginger, berries, mint (optional)

Nutritional Information: Calories: Varies | Protein: Varies | Carbohydrates: Varies | Fat: Varies

Instructions:

1. Brew a strong batch of tea using the tea bags and sugar. Allow it to cool to room temperature.
2. Transfer the tea to a glass jar, leaving some room at the top.
3. Add the SCOBY to the jar.
4. Cover the jar with a breathable cloth and secure it with a rubber band.
5. Allow the kombucha to ferment in a dark, room-temperature place for 7-14 days, depending on taste preference.
6. After fermentation, remove the SCOBY and reserve some liquid as a starter for the next batch.
7. Optional: Add flavorings like ginger, berries, or mint to the kombucha.
8. Bottle the kombucha and refrigerate.

Serving Suggestions:

Serve chilled Kombucha as a fizzy and probiotic-rich drink. Enjoy it as a refreshing beverage on its own or with a slice of lime for added zest.

Golden Milk Latte

Preparation Time: 10 minutes

Serves: 2

Ingredients:

- 2 cups unsweetened almond milk
- 1 teaspoon ground turmeric
- 1/2 teaspoon ground ginger
- 1/4 teaspoon ground cinnamon
- A pinch of black pepper
- 1 teaspoon coconut oil
- Stevia or another sugar-free sweetener to taste (optional)

Nutritional Information: Calories: 40 | Protein: 1g | Carbohydrates: 2g | Fat: 3g

Instructions:

1. In a saucepan, heat almond milk over medium heat until warm but not boiling.
2. Whisk in ground turmeric, ground ginger, ground cinnamon, black pepper, and coconut oil.
3. Continue to whisk until the mixture is well combined and heated through.
4. Sweeten with stevia if desired and adjust to taste.
5. Pour the golden milk into mugs and serve warm.

Serving Suggestions:

Golden Milk Latte is a comforting and anti-inflammatory beverage. Enjoy it in the evening as a soothing alternative to traditional tea or coffee.

Matcha and Green Tea

Preparation Time: 5 minutes

Serves: 1

Ingredients:

- 1 teaspoon matcha powder
- 1 cup hot water (not boiling)

- 1 tablespoon coconut cream or unsweetened almond milk
- Stevia or another sugar-free sweetener to taste (optional)

Nutritional Information: Calories: 5 | Protein: 1g | Carbohydrates: 1g | Fat: 1g

Instructions:

1. In a bowl, sift matcha powder to avoid lumps.
2. Add hot water to the matcha powder and whisk until frothy using a bamboo whisk or a spoon.
3. Heat coconut cream or almond milk until warm but not boiling.
4. Pour the matcha tea into a cup and top with warmed coconut cream or almond milk.
5. Sweeten with stevia if desired and stir well before serving.

Serving Suggestions:

Matcha and Green Tea provide a concentrated source of antioxidants. Enjoy it as a morning ritual or a mid-afternoon pick-me-up for a focused and calm energy boost.

Coconut Water

Preparation Time: N/A

Serves: 1

Ingredients:

- Fresh coconut water from 1 young coconut

Nutritional Information: Calories: 46 | Protein: 2g | Carbohydrates: 9g | Fat: 0g

Instructions:

1. Use a cleaver to carefully open a young coconut.
2. Pour the coconut water into a glass.

Serving Suggestions:

Coconut Water is a natural and hydrating beverage. Enjoy it on its own as a refreshing drink or blend it with berries for a tropical smoothie.

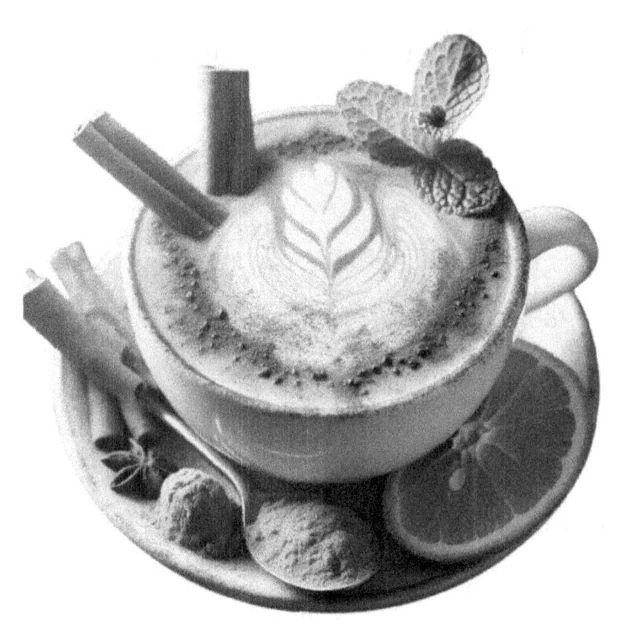

CHAPTER 7

30-Day Meal Sample

Please note that the provided meal plan is a sample and should not be interpreted as a recommendation to consume all the listed recipes in a single day.

This meal plan aims to offer inspiration and guidance for healthy meal preparation. Feel free to customize this plan to suit your preferences and dietary requirements

Day 1:

Breakfast: Coconut Flour Chocolate Chip Cookies

Lunch: Cauliflower Fried Rice

Dinner: Baked Cod with Lemon and Herbs

Snack: Chia Seed Pudding with Berries

Beverage: Moringa Tea

Day 2:

Breakfast: Cinnamon Almond Butter Porridge

Lunch: Turkey Lettuce Wraps

Dinner: Lamb and Buckwheat Meatballs

Snack: Sugar-Free Coconut Yogurt Parfait

Beverage: Cucumber Mint Infused Water

Day 3:

Breakfast: Vanilla Coconut Macaroons

Lunch: Greek Salad with Grilled Chicken

Dinner: Chicken Soup

Snack: Cocoa-Dusted Almonds

Beverage: Golden Milk Latte

Day 4:

Breakfast: Quinoa Breakfast Bowl

Lunch: Zucchini Noodles with Pesto

Dinner: Cabbage Rolls with Turkey and Cauliflower Rice

Snack: Almond Flour Banana Bread

Beverage: Matcha and Green Tea

Day 5:

Breakfast: Coconut Water

Lunch: Millet & Grilled Vegetable Salad

Dinner: Taco Salad

Snack: Berry Herbal Iced Tea

Beverage: Sparkling Ginger Limeade

Day 6:

Breakfast: Zucchini Frittata

Lunch: Salmon and Avocado Lettuce Wraps

Dinner: Paprika Roasted Cabbage Wedges

Snack: Avocado Chocolate Mousse

Beverage: Turmeric Golden Milk Smoothie

Day 7:

Breakfast: Gluten-Free Waffles

Lunch: Stuffed Bell Peppers

Dinner: Cauliflower Hummus

Snack: Coconut Berry Smoothie

Beverage: Hibiscus Ginger Iced Tea

Day 8:

Breakfast: Coconut Flour Chocolate Chip Cookies

Lunch: Quinoa Breakfast Bowl

Dinner: Baked Cod with Lemon and Herbs

Snack: Chia Seed Pudding with Berries

Beverage: Cucumber Mint Infused Water

Day 9:

Breakfast: Cinnamon Almond Butter Porridge

Lunch: Chicken Soup

Dinner: Lamb and Buckwheat Meatballs

Snack: Sugar-Free Coconut Yogurt Parfait

Beverage: Golden Milk Latte

Day 10:

Breakfast: Vanilla Coconut Macaroons

Lunch: Zucchini Noodles with Pesto

Dinner: Cabbage Rolls with Turkey and Cauliflower Rice

Snack: Cocoa-Dusted Almonds

Beverage: Matcha and Green Tea

Day 11:

Breakfast: Quinoa Breakfast Bowl

Lunch: Millet & Grilled Vegetable Salad

Dinner: Taco Salad

Snack: Berry Herbal Iced Tea

Beverage: Sparkling Ginger Limeade

Day 12:

Breakfast: Coconut Water

Lunch: Greek Salad with Grilled Chicken

Dinner: Chicken Soup

Snack: Almond Flour Banana Bread

Beverage: Matcha and Green Tea

Day 13:

Breakfast: Zucchini Frittata

Lunch: Salmon and Avocado Lettuce Wraps

Dinner: Paprika Roasted Cabbage Wedges

Snack: Avocado Chocolate Mousse

Beverage: Turmeric Golden Milk Smoothie

Day 14:

Breakfast: Gluten-Free Waffles

Lunch: Stuffed Bell Peppers

Dinner: Cauliflower Hummus

Snack: Coconut Berry Smoothie

Beverage: Hibiscus Ginger Iced Tea

Day 15:

Breakfast: Coconut Flour Chocolate Chip Cookies

Lunch: Quinoa Breakfast Bowl

Dinner: Baked Cod with Lemon and Herbs

Snack: Chia Seed Pudding with Berries

Beverage: Cucumber Mint Infused Water

Day 16:

Breakfast: Cinnamon Almond Butter Porridge

Lunch: Chicken Soup

Dinner: Lamb and Buckwheat Meatballs

Snack: Sugar-Free Coconut Yogurt Parfait

Beverage: Golden Milk Latte

Day 17:

Breakfast: Vanilla Coconut Macaroons

Lunch: Zucchini Noodles with Pesto

Dinner: Cabbage Rolls with Turkey and Cauliflower Rice

Snack: Cocoa-Dusted Almonds

Beverage: Matcha and Green Tea

Day 18:

Breakfast: Quinoa Breakfast Bowl

Lunch: Millet & Grilled Vegetable Salad

Dinner: Taco Salad

Snack: Berry Herbal Iced Tea

Beverage: Sparkling Ginger Limeade

Day 19:

Breakfast: Coconut Water

Lunch: Greek Salad with Grilled Chicken

Dinner: Chicken Soup

Snack: Almond Flour Banana Bread

Beverage: Matcha and Green Tea

Day 20:

Breakfast: Zucchini Frittata

Lunch: Salmon and Avocado Lettuce Wraps

Dinner: Paprika Roasted Cabbage Wedges

Snack: Avocado Chocolate Mousse

Beverage: Turmeric Golden Milk Smoothie

Day 21:

Breakfast: Gluten-Free Waffles

Lunch: Stuffed Bell Peppers

Dinner: Cauliflower Hummus

Snack: Coconut Berry Smoothie

Beverage: Hibiscus Ginger Iced Tea

Day 22:

Breakfast: Coconut Flour Chocolate Chip Cookies

Lunch: Quinoa Breakfast Bowl

Dinner: Baked Cod with Lemon and Herbs

Snack: Chia Seed Pudding with Berries

Beverage: Cucumber Mint Infused Water

Day 23:

Breakfast: Cinnamon Almond Butter Porridge

Lunch: Chicken Soup

Dinner: Lamb and Buckwheat Meatballs

Snack: Sugar-Free Coconut Yogurt Parfait

Beverage: Golden Milk Latte

Day 24:

Breakfast: Vanilla Coconut Macaroons

Lunch: Zucchini Noodles with Pesto

Dinner: Cabbage Rolls with Turkey and Cauliflower Rice

Snack: Cocoa-Dusted Almonds

Beverage: Matcha and Green Tea

Day 25:

Breakfast: Quinoa Breakfast Bowl

Lunch: Millet & Grilled Vegetable Salad

Dinner: Taco Salad

Snack: Berry Herbal Iced Tea

Beverage: Sparkling Ginger Limeade

Day 26:

Breakfast: Coconut Water

Lunch: Greek Salad with Grilled Chicken

Dinner: Chicken Soup

Snack: Almond Flour Banana Bread

Beverage: Matcha and Green Tea

Day 27:

Breakfast: Zucchini Frittata

Lunch: Salmon and Avocado Lettuce Wraps

Dinner: Paprika Roasted Cabbage Wedges

Snack: Avocado Chocolate Mousse

Beverage: Turmeric Golden Milk Smoothie

Day 28:

Breakfast: Gluten-Free Waffles

Lunch: Stuffed Bell Peppers

Dinner: Cauliflower Hummus

Snack: Coconut Berry Smoothie

Beverage: Hibiscus Ginger Iced Tea

Day 29:

Breakfast: Coconut Flour Chocolate Chip Cookies

Lunch: Quinoa Breakfast Bowl

Dinner: Baked Cod with Lemon and Herbs

Snack: Chia Seed Pudding with Berries

Beverage: Cucumber Mint Infused Water

Day 30:

Breakfast: Cinnamon Almond Butter Porridge

Lunch: Chicken Soup

Dinner: Lamb and Buckwheat Meatballs

Snack: Sugar-Free Coconut Yogurt Parfait

Beverage: Golden Milk Latte

This comprehensive 30-day Anti-Candida Diet Meal Plan offers a diverse range of recipes, ensuring a balanced and enjoyable approach to the dietary guidelines. Adjustments can be made based on personal preferences and nutritional needs.

CHAPTER 8

Conclusion

This Anti-Candida Diet Cookbook is a comprehensive guide to the Anti Candida diet. It includes a detailed explanation of the principles of the diet, the benefits of following it, and a list of foods to eat and avoid.

This book also provides a comprehensive shopping list for the Anti Candida diet, as well as recipes for breakfast, lunch, dinner, desserts, and snacks that are suitable for the diet. The recipes are plant-based, soy-free, corn-free, sugar-free, dairy-free, and gluten-free. This book also includes a 30-day meal plan sample that follows the Anti Candida diet.

The Anti Candida diet is a low-sugar, anti-inflammatory diet that aims to reduce the overgrowth of Candida, a type of yeast that naturally resides in the human body.

The diet is designed to eliminate foods that promote Candida growth, such as sugar, refined carbohydrates, and alcohol, while promoting the consumption of foods that are low in sugar and high in nutrients. By following the Anti Candida diet, you can help restore the balance of gut flora and reduce Candida overgrowth. This can lead to improved digestion, reduced inflammation, increased energy, improved immune function, weight loss, improved skin health, and reduced risk of Candida overgrowth.

The recipes in this cookbook are designed to be nutritious, delicious, and easy to prepare. They are made with simple, whole food ingredients that are easy to find at your local grocery store.

Whether you're new to the Anti Candida diet or you're looking for new recipes to add to your repertoire, this cookbook is an excellent resource to help you achieve your health goals.

Remember to consult with your healthcare provider before starting any new diet or supplement regimen. This Anti Candida Diet Cookbook is not intended to diagnose, treat, cure, or prevent any disease. It is intended to provide information and recipes that can help you improve your health and well-being. I hope this cookbook helps you on your journey to better health.

www.ingramcontent.com/pod-product-compliance
Lightning Source LLC
Chambersburg PA
CBHW060946260726
48661CB00005B/1782